HOLISTIC APPROACHES TO PREVENTING AND MANAGING OSTEOPOROSIS

Expert Guide To Robust Skeletal Health - Integrating Mind, Body, And Nutrition To Prevent And Manage Osteoporosis

DR. CHRIS FRIEDRICH

Disclaimer

This book on Herbal Remedies is intended solely for informational and educational purposes.

The content provided within this book is based on general knowledge and should not be considered as professional advice. The author is not a licensed medical professional, and the information presented here is not intended to diagnose, treat, cure, or prevent any disease.

Readers are advised to consult with qualified healthcare professionals before initiating any herbal remedies or making changes to their existing health regimen. The author and publisher disclaim any responsibility for any adverse effects or consequences resulting from the use of information contained in this book.

It's important to note that the content of this book is not endorsed by any specific platform or affiliated with any product or service.

The author does not receive any compensation or benefits from the promotion of specific herbal products or brands.

Readers should exercise their discretion and judgment when applying the information from this book, and they are encouraged to conduct further research and seek guidance from healthcare professionals to make informed decisions about their health and well-being.

The comprehensive and priceless resource "Holistic Approaches to Preventing and Managing Osteoporosis" covers the many facets of osteoporosis prevention and management.

To lessen the effects of osteoporosis, which is defined as the weakening of bones, a comprehensive understanding and strategy are required. The foundation is laid in the introduction, which emphasizes the value of prevention and takes a comprehensive approach to bone health.

The next chapters explain the construction, makeup, and intricate remodelling process of bones, delving into the complexities of bone anatomy and physiology. The book thoroughly covers genetic predisposition, hormonal impacts, lifestyle, environmental variables, and medical problems associated with osteoporosis since it is important to understand the elements impacting bone health.

In Chapter 3, when the book examines vital elements like calcium, magnesium, and vitamin D and stresses a comprehensive nutritional approach that includes plant-based meals and superfoods, nutrition becomes clear to be a crucial component. Chapter 4 offers an overview of customized physical activities and exercises, including workouts involving weightlifting, strength training, flexibility, and balance.

The lifestyle changes covered in Chapter 5 highlight stress management strategies and the need to get enough sleep, while also illuminating the negative impacts of smoking and binge drinking. After that, the book discusses evidence-based methods for integrating herbal and natural supplements with traditional medical therapies.

In Chapter 7, the mind-body link is discussed in detail, with topics including stress and cortisol levels, mindfulness exercises, meditation, and the advantages of yoga for bone health. In Chapter 8, integrative medicine and holistic healthcare practitioners are covered, with a focus on working together with experts.

The discussion of preventative techniques is expanded in Chapters 9 and 10, with a focus on bone health from childhood through menopause and beyond.

The book ends with case studies and success stories that demonstrate how holistic methods may be applied in real-world situations and bolster the effectiveness of the tactics covered.

To sum up, "Holistic Approaches to Preventing and Managing Osteoporosis" offers individuals useful advice on how to take control of their bone health in addition to synthesizing scientific information on the condition.

The book provides readers with a full toolset for managing and preventing osteoporosis by using a holistic approach, which makes it a valuable resource in the field of bone health literature.

Overview

Osteoporosis is a serious public health issue that is defined by the loss of bone mass and density, which raises the risk of fractures. Osteoporosis is becoming more common as the world's population ages, which calls for a comprehensive and all-encompassing strategy to manage and prevent the disorder. Through a holistic perspective, this book examines several elements of osteoporosis prevention and management, taking into account not just conventional medical therapies but also lifestyle choices, dietary habits, and psychological characteristics that are linked to bone health.

Knowing What Osteoporosis Is Meaning And Reasons

A skeletal illness called osteoporosis is characterized by the weakening of the bones, which puts people at higher risk of fractures. Since the disorder frequently shows no symptoms until a fracture happens, early identification and preventative care are essential.

An imbalance in bone remodeling, when bone resorption surpasses bone production, is one of the main causes of osteoporosis. Age, hormonal fluctuations (especially in postmenopausal women), genetics, and lifestyle decisions like smoking and sedentary behavior can all be blamed for this imbalance.

It is essential to comprehend the complex etiology of osteoporosis to develop effective preventative measures.

The Value Of Prevention

Osteoporosis affects people differently, and prevention is key to lessening its effects on people and healthcare systems. Osteoporosis-related fractures have a significant financial cost and a profoundly negative emotional impact on those who experience them. Preventive measures improve the quality of life for people who are at risk overall and allow for more effective resource allocation. Moreover, by lowering the incidence of fractures and their related sequelae, prophylaxis eases the burden on healthcare systems. The value of prevention goes beyond lowering the risk of fractures; it also includes preserving general bone health, which is essential for a person's freedom and mobility.

An All-Encompassing View On Bone Health

Beyond the confines of the conventional medical model, a holistic approach to bone health takes into account a multitude of factors that impact skeletal health. This method acknowledges that lifestyle decisions, dietary habits, and mental health all have an impact on bone health in addition to hormonal and hereditary predispositions. The goal of holistic treatments is to develop a complete plan that tackles the underlying causes of osteoporosis while taking into account the interconnection of these variables.

Interventions In Lifestyle Engagement In Exercise

The foundation of a comprehensive strategy for managing and preventing osteoporosis is regular physical exercise. Strength and bone density are enhanced by weight-bearing activities, resistance training, and balance-enhancing exercises. Weight-bearing activities like dancing, running, and walking promote the growth of new bone and lower the risk of fractures. Resistance exercise also increases muscle mass, and since it improves general strength and coordination, it indirectly helps bone health. A holistic viewpoint emphasizes the necessity for individualized exercise plans based on an individual's age, fitness level, and particular risk factors to acknowledge the symbiotic link between physical activity and bone health.

Giving Up Smoking And Moderate Drinking

Lifestyle decisions including smoking and binge drinking have been associated with a higher risk of osteoporosis. Smoking interferes with the generation of hormones necessary for healthy bones, which has a detrimental impact on bone density. In a similar vein, consuming too much alcohol can upset the delicate balance between bone growth and resorption.

To lower the risk of osteoporosis, a comprehensive approach promotes alcohol use in moderation and smoking cessation programs. Through the treatment of these modifiable risk factors, people may take an active role in their bone health.

Dietary Considerations Vitamin D And Calcium

Bone health is greatly influenced by nutrition, and a holistic approach views getting enough calcium and vitamin D as critical components of preventative measures. A lack of calcium can affect bone density since it is a vital component of bones. Vitamin D is essential for bone mineralization and helps the body absorb calcium. Promoting a well-balanced diet full of dairy products, leafy green vegetables, and fortified foods is an important part of holistic therapies. Furthermore, an all-encompassing nutritional strategy for osteoporosis prevention must include adequate exposure to sunshine, a natural source of vitamin D.

Micronutrients And Nutrient Synergy

A holistic dietary approach acknowledges the significance of nutrient synergy and takes into account the impact of other micronutrients in bone health, in addition to calcium and vitamin D. Bone mineralization and metabolism are aided by trace minerals such copper and zinc, magnesium, phosphorus, and vitamin K. For optimal bone health, a diet rich in a range of nutrients in sufficient levels is recommended.

To guarantee a full spectrum of vital nutrients needed for preserving bone density and preventing osteoporosis, holistic dietary guidelines place a strong emphasis on consuming a varied variety of foods.

Psychosocial Elements

<u>Stress Reduction</u>

Stress and mental health are examples of psychosocial elements that are becoming more widely acknowledged as influences on bone health. Prolonged stress can cause hormone abnormalities that impact bone remodeling and raise the risk of osteoporosis. Integrating stress-reduction methods like mindfulness, meditation, and relaxation exercises into prophylactic plans is part of a holistic approach. People can improve the effectiveness of other preventative actions and establish a supportive environment for bone health by addressing psychological variables.

Social Support And Life Quality

Quality of life and social support are essential elements of a comprehensive strategy for osteoporosis prevention. Having a fulfilling life and solid social ties may have a great impact on one's general well-being, which includes bone health. Studies have connected social isolation and loneliness to negative health outcomes; a holistic approach acknowledges the value of social relationships in promoting mental and physical well-being. Taking part in joyful and fulfilling activities enhances a person's resilience overall and may indirectly promote bone health through healthy lifestyle choices.

A thorough grasp of the variables affecting bone health is essential to preventing and treating osteoporosis holistically. Each idea contributes to the creation of a complex plan that goes beyond conventional medical procedures, from the definition and causes of osteoporosis to the significance of prevention. Together, individuals, politicians, and healthcare professionals may promote bone health throughout an individual's lifetime by adopting a holistic viewpoint.

A holistic approach recognizes the interconnection of lifestyle modifications, dietary considerations, and psychological variables as the pillars of treatment. Osteoporosis prevention is becoming more and more important as the world's population ages, and a comprehensive approach offers a path forward for practical and long-lasting solutions to this widespread public health concern.

CHAPTER ONE
BONE PHYSIOLOGY AND ANATOMY

The human skeleton, a wonder of biological engineering, forms the body's structure, supporting critical organs, allowing for mobility, and giving structural support. The basic building blocks of this system, bones, are dynamic structures with intricate anatomies and physiologies. Living tissue, minerals, and collagen fibers combine to produce the matrix that gives bones their strength and durability. The special characteristics of bone tissue are a result of the complex interactions between minerals, proteins, and cells.

Bone Composition And Structure:

Bones' complex composition determines their structural stability. The two types of bone tissues that make up bones are trabecular (spongy) and cortical (compact), each with unique properties. The thick and strong cortical bone is found in the outer layer, whereas the more flexible trabecular bone is found in the interior sections.

The main components of the extracellular matrix that give bones their stiffness are hydroxyapatite crystals, calcium, and phosphate. A dynamic equilibrium between hardness and flexibility is created by the woven collagen fibers into this matrix, which improves tensile strength and is crucial for bone function.

The Process Of Bone Remodelling

To keep bones healthy and adjust to mechanical pressures, bone remodeling is a dynamic, ongoing process. It includes the coordinated actions of osteoblasts and osteoclasts, which are the specific cells in charge of creating and resorbing bone, respectively. While osteoblasts go on to build new bone matrix, osteoclasts degrade damaged or aging bone tissue, releasing minerals into the blood.

This complex dance keeps the skeletal system's structural integrity intact by promoting bone regeneration and repair and limiting the buildup of microdamage.

Affecting Factors For Bone Health

Understanding the many elements that intimately affect bone health is essential to managing and preventing osteoporosis. Genetic factors are important since a person's susceptibility to bone disorders might run in the family. Bone mineralization is largely dependent on dietary variables, particularly calcium and vitamin D consumption. Exercise that involves lifting weights, in particular, promotes bone remodeling and increases bone density. Hormonal balance has a major influence on bone health, particularly throughout menopause and puberty. Furthermore, bad lifestyle decisions like smoking and binge drinking can hurt bone density.

Holistic Methods For Osteoporosis Management And Prevention

Osteoporosis must be prevented and managed using a multifaceted strategy that takes into account all aspects of bone health. Nutrition is important; a balanced diet full of calcium, vitamin D, and other important nutrients is recommended. Strong and mineralized bones are supported by the consumption of these nutrients. Frequent exercise that includes strength training and weightlifting improves bone density and skeletal health in general.

A comprehensive strategy also includes lifestyle changes as a crucial component. Given that smoking has been connected to lower bone density and a higher risk of fractures, quitting is imperative. It is best to consume alcohol in moderation since too much alcohol might harm your bones. Furthermore, it's critical to maintain a healthy body weight because obesity and underweight can both reduce bone density.

Hormonal balance is an important factor, especially for women who are getting close to menopause. In certain situations, hormone replacement treatment (HRT) may be advised to lessen the impact of hormonal fluctuations on bone density. On an individual basis, nevertheless, one should carefully weigh the advantages and disadvantages of HRT.

Frequent evaluations of bone density using techniques such as dual-energy X-ray absorptiometry (DEXA) scans are necessary for osteoporosis early identification and tracking. Timely execution of preventative measures and suitable medical treatment is made possible by early intervention. Healthcare providers may prescribe pharmaceutical treatments, such as bisphosphonates, hormone therapy, and bone-forming drugs, based on a patient's unique risk factors and bone health status.

Education campaigns that focus on osteoporosis risk factors, preventative treatments, and the significance of lifestyle changes are essential. At the societal level, public health campaigns and community engagement initiatives help to promote a proactive attitude to bone health.

The development and use of holistic methods for osteoporosis prevention and management require a thorough grasp of the anatomy and physiology of bones as well as an awareness of the variables impacting bone health. People may actively contribute to the maintenance of bone health and lower the risk of osteoporotic fractures by addressing diet, lifestyle, hormonal balance, and medicinal treatments. This will provide a greater quality of life as they age.

CHAPTER TWO
OSTEOPOROSIS RISK FACTORS

Reduced bone density and microarchitectural degradation of bone tissue, which increases fragility and fracture risk, are the hallmarks of osteoporosis, a complex skeletal condition. Developing comprehensive strategies to prevent and treat osteoporosis requires an understanding of the risk factors linked to the illness.

Molecular Predisposition

The risk of osteoporosis in an individual is mostly determined by genetic factors. Certain genetic variants and indicators have been linked by research to fracture risk and bone density.

Genetic variations affecting bone metabolism are more likely to be inherited by those with a family history of osteoporosis. Researching the hereditary susceptibility to osteoporosis offers important insights into the molecular processes that maintain healthy bones. Personalized therapies to reduce the risk of osteoporosis in vulnerable individuals may be provided via preventative measures tailored according to genetic profile.

Hormonal Effects

Hormonal variables have a significant impact on bone health, especially sex hormones like testosterone and estrogen. Because it prevents bone resorption, estrogen in particular is essential for preserving bone density. Osteoporosis risk increases and bone loss is hastened in postmenopausal women due to a decrease in estrogen levels. Men's hormonal changes, such as declining testosterone levels with age, also have a role in bone loss. Strategies that treat hormonal imbalances through lifestyle changes, hormone replacement therapy, or other focused interventions should be taken into account in holistic approaches to osteoporosis prevention.

Environmental And Lifestyle Factors

The onset and advancement of osteoporosis are mostly influenced by environmental factors and lifestyle decisions. Poor diet, particularly in terms of calcium and vitamin D consumption, can harm bones. Reduced bone density is a result of sedentary lifestyles and insufficient weight-bearing activity. The metabolism of bone is negatively impacted by smoking and binge drinking, which raises the risk of fractures.

To maximize bone health across the lifespan, comprehensive measures must be put into practice. These include encouraging a bone-friendly lifestyle that includes a balanced diet, frequent exercise, and abstaining from bad habits.

Medical Disorders Associated With Osteoporosis

Osteoporosis risk is raised by specific medical conditions and therapies. The delicate balance of bone remodeling can be upset by chronic illnesses such as rheumatoid arthritis, inflammatory bowel disease, and endocrine disorders, which can result in bone loss. Osteoporosis can also result from long-term usage of drugs like glucocorticoids, which are frequently used for inflammatory diseases. The integration of care for underlying medical diseases, tailoring medication regimens to reduce bone-related adverse effects, and including efforts to enhance bone health in patients with chronic illnesses are all important components of holistic approaches to osteoporosis prevention and therapy.

Holistic Methods For Osteoporosis Management And Prevention

Osteoporosis prevention and management necessitate a thorough and integrated strategy that takes into account the various aspects affecting bone health. To reduce risk factors and improve overall skeletal health, a holistic approach includes dietary treatments, focused exercise programs, tailored healthcare plans, and lifestyle adjustments.

Interventions Related To Nutrition

A comprehensive strategy for treating osteoporosis must include modifying diet to promote bone health. A sufficient consumption of calcium and vitamin D is necessary for the mineralization of bones. To achieve ideal bone density, a well-balanced diet full of dairy, almonds, leafy green vegetables, and fortified foods can be included. Supplemental nutrients could also be advised for those who are susceptible to deficiencies.

A comprehensive approach to osteoporosis prevention must take into account the particular needs of each patient and customize dietary therapies accordingly, correcting any deficits.

Physical Activity And Exercise

Exercises that include weight-bearing and resistance are essential parts of a comprehensive strategy to prevent osteoporosis. Frequent exercise promotes the growth of new bones and preserves bone mass. Walking, running, and weight training are examples of weight-bearing workouts that are very beneficial for maintaining bone health. Exercise regimens should be customized for each person based on their talents and interests, taking age, degree of fitness, and general health into consideration. A physically active lifestyle and the incorporation of exercise into everyday activities are important components of the comprehensive therapy of osteoporosis.

Techniques For Preventing Falls

Since fractures from falls are a major risk for people with osteoporosis, fall prevention techniques must be a part of holistic treatment plans.

Fall risk can be decreased by making changes to the surrounding environment, such as eliminating trip hazards at home, adding handrails, and upgrading lighting. Exercises for balance and coordination are important parts of fall prevention plans. Healthcare professionals are essential in teaching people the value of preventing falls and offering advice on how to create safe living spaces.

Hormone Replacement Treatment

Hormonal changes in postmenopausal women haveten the loss of bone. In certain cases, hormone replacement therapy (HRT) can be viewed as a component of a comprehensive strategy for controlling osteoporosis. On the other hand, choosing to get HRT should be the result of a careful evaluation of the advantages and disadvantages, taking into account each person's preferences and state of health. Optimizing bone health while reducing potential adverse effects requires regular monitoring of hormone levels and corresponding medication adjustments. Informed people and healthcare professionals must work together to integrate HRT into a comprehensive care plan.

Drug-Related Interventions

Pharmacological therapies can be required in some circumstances to properly control osteoporosis. Antiresorptive drugs, such as denosumab and bisphosphonates, can slow down bone turnover and stop more bone loss. In some circumstances, anabolic drugs such as teriparatide, which promote bone growth, may be taken into consideration. However, each patient should receive customized treatment when using pharmaceutical treatments, taking into consideration variables including comorbidities, fracture risk, and possible adverse effects.

To maximize overall results, holistic treatment entails striking a balance between pharmaceutical and non-pharmacological therapies.

Patient Empowerment And Education

Prioritizing patient education and empowerment is crucial in holistic approaches to osteoporosis prevention and treatment. Giving people thorough knowledge about risk factors, preventative strategies, and bone health improves their capacity to make wise lifestyle decisions. Encouraging patients to take an active role in their care includes encouraging self-management techniques, encouraging patients to follow their treatment regimens, and ensuring honest communication between patients and healthcare professionals. Outreach campaigns for the community might incorporate educational initiatives that highlight the significance of bone health for a variety of demographics.

Multidisciplinary Cooperation

Healthcare practitioners must collaborate collaboratively to address the complicated nature of osteoporosis.

To create complete treatment plans, orthopedic experts, endocrinologists, dietitians, physical therapists, and primary care physicians should work together. A comprehensive evaluation of each person is possible with a multidisciplinary approach, which takes into account both skeletal and general health. A more successful and comprehensive approach to osteoporosis prevention and management is promoted by coordinated care, which guarantees that interventions and preventative measures are tailored to the specific needs of each patient.

a comprehensive understanding of the various risk factors affecting bone health is essential to managing and preventing osteoporosis.

The complex terrain of osteoporosis includes genetic predisposition, hormonal impacts, lifestyle and environmental variables, and medical diseases. Nutritional therapies, physical activity and exercise, fall prevention, hormone replacement therapy, pharmaceutical interventions, patient education, and interdisciplinary teamwork are all included in a holistic approach. Healthcare professionals may maximize osteoporosis prevention and management by addressing these factors holistically, individualized treatment plans, and long-term bone health.

CHAPTER THREE
BONE HEALTH NUTRITION

Osteoporosis is a disorder marked by weakening bones and an increased risk of fractures. Nutrition is crucial to the prevention and management of this illness. This comprehensive approach emphasizes the need for essential nutrients for strong bones, with particular attention paid to calcium, vitamin D, and magnesium.

As a vital mineral for bone strength and structure, calcium is essential to maintaining the health of bones. Getting enough calcium is important all through life, but it's especially important throughout childhood and adolescence when bone growth is at its highest. Fortified meals, leafy greens, and dairy products are great sources of calcium. But reaching the right amounts of calcium requires more than simply supply; other elements like bioavailability and the way other nutrients are balanced out also matter in promoting healthy bone mineralization.

Another essential vitamin that has a major impact on bone health is vitamin D. Maintaining appropriate serum calcium and phosphate levels and controlling calcium absorption are its key responsibilities. Common sources of vitamin D include sun exposure, supplements, and foods fortified with vitamin D. When it comes to preventing osteoporosis, it is essential to make sure that one has enough amounts of vitamin D, particularly in areas with little sunshine or in those who spend less time in the sun. Since calcium and vitamin D interact fundamentally, a thorough dietary strategy is needed.

Often overlooked in favor of calcium and vitamin D, magnesium is becoming more and more recognized for its role in maintaining healthy bones. It contributes to overall skeletal integrity by influencing bone mineral density and bone crystal formation.

A healthy diet should include foods high in magnesium, such as green vegetables, whole grains, nuts, and seeds.

The complicated interplay of dietary interactions in preserving ideal bone health is highlighted by the delicate link among calcium, vitamin D, and magnesium.

Beyond specific dietary supplements, a comprehensive dietary strategy is crucial for managing and preventing osteoporosis. Plant-based diets, which prioritize the intake of fruits, vegetables, legumes, and whole grains, are becoming more and more popular.

Numerous vitamins, minerals, and phytonutrients found in these diets all work together to support bone health. Many plant-based diets have an alkaline quality that is thought to balance the acidic by-products of animal protein digestion, potentially maintaining bone health. Furthermore, plant-based diets' anti-inflammatory and antioxidant qualities may help bone health indirectly by reducing chronic inflammation, which is linked to bone resorption.

Superfoods, known for their high nutritional content, are becoming more and more acknowledged for their ability to support bone health. Examples include leafy greens high in vitamin K, which is essential for bone metabolism, and fatty fish high in omega-3 fatty acids, which may help with bone density. Due to their high antioxidant content, berries, nuts, and seeds can also be included in a diet that is beneficial to bones. Superfoods are part of a more comprehensive holistic approach that recognizes the complementary roles of different nutrients on bone health.

a comprehensive strategy for treating and preventing osteoporosis necessitates a sophisticated comprehension of dietary habits, critical nutrients, and the mutually reinforcing relationships between diverse elements. Maintaining the strength of your bones requires taking care of your core components, which include magnesium, calcium, and vitamin D. Moreover, plant-based diets and the addition of superfoods are examples of holistic dietary strategies that offer a wide range of nutrients that work together to promote good bone health.

A comprehensive approach is becoming more and more necessary in the quest for skeletal well-being as research reveals the complex relationships between diet and bone metabolism.

CHAPTER FOUR
EXERCISE AND PHYSICAL ACTIVITY IN

Exercise and physical activity are essential for managing and preventing osteoporosis, a disorder marked by weakening bones and a higher risk of fractures. Maintaining bone density, muscular strength, and general physical function requires frequent physical activity. Exercises involving weight bearing, including dancing, running, and walking, are very good for your bones.

By encouraging bone growth and halting bone loss, these activities lower the risk of osteoporosis-related fractures. Increased bone density and strength result from weight-bearing activities because they put mechanical stress on the bones and encourage the growth of osteoblasts, the cells that make new bone.

Exercises that involve bearing weight on the body are categorized as weight-bearing exercises because they need the bones to sustain the weight of the body. This includes jogging, walking, hiking, and aerobic workouts. Because these activities put the bones under mechanical strain, which causes them to adapt and become denser, they are very helpful in boosting bone health. Exercises involving weight bearing have been shown to improve bone mineral density (BMD), which is essential for avoiding osteoporosis. Including these exercises in a regular fitness regimen is crucial for those who want to strengthen their bones and lower their chance of osteoporosis-related fractures.

Another essential element of a comprehensive strategy for preventing osteoporosis is strength training, which consists of resistance exercises that focus on building muscle mass and strength. Although bone mineral density may not be directly affected by these workouts, overall bone health is greatly enhanced by them. Muscles under stress from strength training apply force to the corresponding bones. Mechanical stress increases bone strength and durability by inducing bone remodeling. Weightlifting, squats, lunges, and other resistance exercises employing weights, resistance bands, or body weight can be customized to a person's level of fitness. Strength training enhances weight-bearing exercises in an exercise program, supporting overall musculoskeletal health.

Exercises for balance and flexibility are crucial parts of a comprehensive strategy for preventing osteoporosis. These workouts, which include tai chi and yoga, target improving balance, flexibility, and coordination. Exercises for flexibility and balance are essential for lowering the risk of falls and fractures in people with osteoporosis, even if they may not have a direct effect on bone density. Stretching activities that increase flexibility help to improve joint mobility and general functional fitness. Additionally, by improving stability and proprioception, balancing exercises reduce the risk of falls. People who are susceptible to fractures from osteoporosis might greatly benefit from including these exercises in a comprehensive fitness regimen.

Personalized exercise programs are a cornerstone of a comprehensive strategy for managing and preventing osteoporosis. Age, degree of fitness, and any pre-existing medical issues are among the particular factors that are specific to each individual. Exercise regimens should thus be tailored to each person's demands and abilities. A thorough examination that takes into account bone density measurements and general health should direct the creation of a suitable workout program. When designing workouts, it's important to take into account things like comorbidities, prior fractures, and individual preferences. With a customized strategy, people may exercise safely and effectively, reducing the chance of injury and optimizing the advantages for bone health.

It is essential to take a comprehensive approach to osteoporosis management and prevention through exercise and physical activity to preserve bone health and lower the risk of fractures. Weight-bearing activities that put mechanical stress on the bones, such as running and walking, increase bone density. Strength training contributes to the resilience and strength of bones by improving overall musculoskeletal health.

Exercises that improve flexibility and balance, such as tai chi and yoga, are essential for osteoporosis patients to avoid fractures and falls. Exercise programs should be customized to each person's needs, taking into consideration age, fitness level, and pre-existing medical concerns, to guarantee a safe and individualized approach. For those at risk of osteoporosis, including these ideas in a thorough fitness program is crucial to enhancing bone health and general well-being.

CHAPTER FIVE
ADJUSTMENTS TO LIFESTYLE
The Effects Of Smoking On Bone Health

An essential component of managing and preventing osteoporosis is understanding the connection between smoking and bone health. Because smoking hurts bone metabolism, it is a substantial risk factor for osteoporosis. It has been demonstrated that nicotine and other dangerous ingredients in tobacco smoke obstruct the absorption of calcium, a crucial mineral for preserving bone density. Additionally, smoking is linked to a higher generation of free radicals, which causes oxidative stress and can aggravate bone loss. Furthermore, smoking has been connected to hormonal abnormalities, namely a reduction in estrogen levels in both men and women, which speeds up the resorption of bone.

Thus, implementing smoking cessation techniques is essential to any comprehensive strategy for managing and preventing osteoporosis.

Drinking Of Alcohol

In the context of osteoporosis prevention, alcohol consumption's effect on bone health is a complex factor to take into account. While there may be some cardiovascular advantages to moderate alcohol use, excessive and long-term alcohol use has been linked to a higher risk of osteoporosis. Alcohol inhibits the creation of osteoblasts, the cells that create bones, and interferes with the absorption of calcium and vitamin D.

In addition to its detrimental effects on the endocrine system, chronic alcohol use also causes hormonal imbalances that exacerbate bone loss. Personalized treatments to address underlying issues contributing to excessive drinking and education on the necessity of moderation in alcohol use should thus be part of a holistic strategy for managing and preventing osteoporosis.

Techniques For Stress Management

An essential component of the comprehensive strategy for managing and preventing osteoporosis is stress management. It is well-recognized that prolonged stress affects bone health via several physiological mechanisms. Increased bone resorption and reduced bone production have been related to elevated levels of stress hormones, such as cortisol. Furthermore, long-term stress can result in unhealthy coping strategies like eating poorly and exercising less, both of which exacerbate bone loss. Using stress-reduction strategies like yoga, meditation, and mindfulness-based stress reduction might lessen the damaging effects of ongoing stress on bone health.

These methods not only assist general well-being and relaxation, but they also create an atmosphere that is favorable for preserving ideal bone density.

The Value Of Good Sleep

Getting enough sleep is a crucial but sometimes disregarded part of managing and preventing osteoporosis holistically. The body goes through critical bone metabolism activities, such as bone growth and repair, while you sleep.

Sleep disturbances, such as insomnia or insufficient sleep duration, can negatively impact these mechanisms and result in weakened bone structure. Lack of sleep has been associated with elevated cortisol levels, which in turn promote bone resorption. Moreover, deep sleep stages are when growth hormone, which is necessary for bone development and maintenance, is released. Thus, a key component of the holistic care of osteoporosis is stressing the need to develop sound sleep habits and treat sleep problems.

Education campaigns should emphasize the relationship between bone health and sleep quality, motivating people to focus and improve their sleep schedules for their general well-being.

a comprehensive strategy for treating and preventing osteoporosis includes addressing a range of lifestyle variables that influence bone health. Important elements of this strategy include quitting smoking, using alcohol in moderation, managing stress, and placing a high priority on getting enough sleep. Creating successful therapies requires an understanding of the complex interactions between these lifestyle variables and bone metabolism. The holistic management of osteoporosis can be greatly aided by personalized counseling, educational campaigns, and the incorporation of these ideas into standard medical procedures. This will ultimately improve the quality of life for those who are either at risk for developing osteoporosis or who have already been diagnosed with it.

CHAPTER SIX
SUPPLEMENTS MADE NATURALLY AND HERBAL

Low bone mass and microarchitectural degradation of bone tissue are the hallmarks of osteoporosis, a systemic skeletal condition that increases bone fragility and fracture risk.

A rising number of people are interested in comprehensive methods of managing and preventing osteoporosis. These methods cover a broad spectrum of tactics, such as dietary adjustments, complementary and alternative medicine, and lifestyle changes.

Herbal and natural supplements have garnered interest as possible means of promoting bone health among them. We will explore the many facets of holistic therapies for osteoporosis in this extensive talk, with an emphasis on herbal and natural supplements.

Synopsis Of Herbal Treatments

For ages, traditional medical systems throughout the world have used herbal treatments to treat a variety of health concerns, including disorders relating to the bones. Herbs are frequently sought for their ability to improve general skeletal health, decrease bone resorption, and increase bone density in the setting of osteoporosis.

Common herbs for supporting bone strength include horsetail (Equisetum arvense), which has a high silica content and has been used historically. Furthermore, it's thought that certain herbs, such as black cohosh (Actaea racemosa) and red clover (Trifolium pratense), contain estrogenic properties that may affect bone metabolism. However, it is important to take caution while using herbal medicines, taking into account individual differences in reaction and the requirement for thorough scientific proof.

Supplements With Supporting Evidence

A crucial element of the comprehensive care of osteoporosis is the integration of supplements based on scientific data. The maintenance of healthy bones depends heavily on calcium and vitamin D, which is especially crucial for preventing osteoporosis. Calcium is essential for the structural integrity of bones, and vitamin D helps the body absorb and use calcium.

The metabolism of bones is also influenced by trace minerals including copper and zinc, magnesium, and vitamin K. Omega-3 fatty acid-containing fish oil supplements have been investigated for possible anti-inflammatory benefits on bone tissue.

The scientific literature on these supplements offers important information on their safety and effectiveness, helping patients and healthcare professionals make well-informed decisions about whether or not to include them in comprehensive osteoporosis management programs.

Combining Conventional Treatments With Holistic Approaches

Integrating holistic methods with traditional therapies is a new paradigm in the therapy of osteoporosis. When treating problems with bone density, conventional therapies including hormone replacement therapy and bisphosphonates are frequently used.

Holistic methods, on the other hand, acknowledge the significance of a comprehensive plan that extends beyond medication treatments. The goal of combining herbal and natural supplements with medical therapies is to maximize the benefits of many therapeutic modalities working in concert.

A tailored strategy is used to lead this integration, taking into account the unique profiles, preferences, and reaction patterns of each patient. Although holistic methods promote general health, it is critical to keep lines of communication open between patients and healthcare professionals to guarantee the security and effectiveness of coordinated therapies.

holistic methods of managing and preventing osteoporosis provide a thorough outlook that goes beyond traditional medication treatments.

With their origins in conventional therapy, herbal and natural supplements offer exciting potential for promoting bone health.

To support clinical practice and assist people in making decisions, a critical assessment of the available data is necessary. Supplements with scientific backing, such as those high in calcium, vitamin D, and other micronutrients, are essential for maintaining bone health. One potential path to improving osteoporosis care is the fusion of holistic methods with traditional therapies.

To achieve the best possible outcomes for individuals who are affected by or at risk of osteoporosis, a collaborative and patient-centered approach is still essential as research into the intricacies of bone metabolism and the effects of holistic therapies continues.

CHAPTER SEVEN
THE MIND-BODY LINK

A key idea in the holistic approach to managing and preventing osteoporosis is the mind-body link. This idea highlights the complex interrelationship between physical and mental health, recognizing that bone health is greatly influenced by mental health. Osteoporosis can develop and worsen as a result of stress, worry, and other psychological causes. Scholars have delved into the processes by which stress impacts bone health, uncovering the part that stress hormones like cortisol play in bone metabolism. Developing holistic approaches to osteoporosis care and prevention requires an understanding of the mind-body relationship.

Stress And Levels Of Cortisol

The main hormone released in reaction to stress, cortisol, has been linked to osteoporosis and has been recognized as a possible risk factor for the condition.

Reduced bone density and poor bone production have been linked to elevated cortisol levels, which can arise from long-term stress. Prolonged stress can also exacerbate the risk of osteoporosis by promoting bad lifestyle choices including poor eating habits and inactivity.

A comprehensive approach to osteoporosis prevention must investigate stress-reduction strategies and treatments, among other interventions, to control and lower stress levels.

Mindfulness And Meditation Techniques

Although mindfulness and meditation have become well-known for their beneficial impacts on mental health, osteoporosis research is beginning to show interest in these practices' possible implications on bone health. According to studies, practicing mindfulness and meditation daily may help control cortisol levels by modifying the stress response. These methods could improve bone health by encouraging a calmer mental state. Furthermore, mindfulness-based therapies have the potential to improve self-awareness, which in turn promotes healthier lifestyle choices.

These choices include better eating habits and greater physical exercise, both of which are essential for managing and preventing osteoporosis.

Yoga And The Health Of Your Bones

Yoga has gained popularity as a comprehensive strategy for supporting bone health. It is an age-old discipline that combines physical postures, breath control, and meditation. Weight-bearing bones are the focus of some yoga postures, which also stimulate bone remodeling and increase bone density. It is well-recognized that weight-bearing activities are good for bone health, and yoga offers a low-impact but efficient way to meet this goal. Furthermore, yoga's mind-body component lowers stress, which may lessen one of the psychological variables associated with osteoporosis. Including yoga in complete programs to prevent osteoporosis provides a holistic approach that takes into account the mental and physical elements of bone health.

the holistic approach to osteoporosis management and prevention acknowledges the complex interactions between the body and mind. Creating complete methods requires an understanding of how stress, cortisol levels, and the potential benefits of yoga and mindfulness practices affect bone health. Healthcare providers may provide patients with more sophisticated and successful therapies that go beyond conventional methods by addressing the mind-body link, which will enhance overall well-being in addition to stronger bones.

CHAPTER EIGHT
PROVIDERS OF HOLISTIC HEALTHCARE

The idea of holistic healthcare providers in osteoporosis prevention and management stems from the understanding that treating this illness calls for an all-encompassing strategy that takes into account the connections between different facets of health. Rather than focusing just on treating osteoporosis symptoms, holistic healthcare providers address the full person, frequently including professionals from other disciplines. This method acknowledges that osteoporosis involves a variety of elements, including genetics, diet, lifestyle, and mental health, in addition to the skeletal system. Physicians, dietitians, physical therapists, mental health specialists, and practitioners of alternative medicine are examples of holistic providers that collaborate to provide customized treatment regimens that are comprehensive.

Complementary And Alternative Medicine

Integrative medicine is essential to the comprehensive strategy for managing and preventing osteoporosis. It entails integrating evidence-based complementary therapies with traditional medical treatments, with a focus on the physical, emotional, and spiritual well-being of the patient. Integrative medicine may combine pharmacological therapies, dietary modifications, exercise routines, and mind-body techniques to treat osteoporosis. For example, enhancing general bone health can be achieved by combining conventional medical therapies with acupuncture, yoga, or meditation. Integrative medicine aims to maximize the benefits of therapies while reducing any negative effects, acknowledging the importance of several therapeutic methods.

Consulting And Working Together With Experts

A comprehensive strategy for osteoporosis therapy and prevention must include specialized advice and teamwork. Experts with specialized knowledge include endocrinologists, rheumatologists, orthopedic surgeons, dietitians, and physical therapists. For example, endocrinologists can treat hormone abnormalities that could lead to bone loss, and orthopedic surgeons can offer advice on surgical procedures if fractures develop. When creating individualized meal regimens high in calcium and vitamin D, which are critical for bone health, nutritionists are invaluable. By creating workout plans that improve bone density and lower the risk of falls, physical therapists make a positive contribution. These professionals work together to guarantee a thorough grasp of the patient's situation, which results in solutions that are more individualized and successful.

The complex nature of osteoporosis is highlighted by the holistic approaches to treating and preventing the disease, which include integrative medicine, holistic healthcare practitioners, and specialist consulting. By adopting a holistic viewpoint that considers an individual's physical, mental, and lifestyle factors, medical professionals can increase the effectiveness of treatments and raise the general quality of life for patients with osteoporosis. In the field of bone health, this integrated and cooperative approach signifies a paradigm change toward patient-centered treatment by highlighting the significance of individualized, evidence-based methods for managing and preventing osteoporosis.

CHAPTER NINE
PREVENTION METHODS THROUGHOUT LIFE

A thorough and all-encompassing strategy for prevention is required for osteoporosis, a crippling skeletal illness marked by decreased bone density and an increased susceptibility to fractures, throughout the lifespan. The preventative measures address the distinct risks and problems that are specific to each period of life.

Bone Health In Childhood And Adolescence

Childhood and adolescence provide the groundwork for bone health, making this time crucial for avoiding osteoporosis in later life. Optimizing peak bone mass acquisition requires regular physical activity, adequate calcium and vitamin D consumption, and both. Strong, thick bones are developed with proper diet, especially during growth spurts.

For children and adolescents to develop lifetime behaviors related to bone health, education, and awareness campaigns that support healthy lifestyle choices—such as a balanced diet and regular exercise—are essential.

Senior And Adult Bone Health

As people enter maturity and later life stages, the emphasis changes to preserving bone health and reducing the causes that lead to bone loss. Maintaining bone density becomes more dependent on weight-bearing activities, strength training, and balance-enhancing exercises.

The foundation of health is still nutrition, with a focus on getting enough calcium, vitamin D, and other important nutrients. Making lifestyle changes, including quitting smoking and drinking less alcohol, is essential for halting the degradation of bones. Individual risk profiles may dictate the need for timely action, such as the use of supplements or pharmaceuticals, in addition to routine bone density tests.

Changes In Hormones During Menopause

Menopause causes substantial hormonal changes, most notably a drop in estrogen levels, which increases the risk of bone loss in women.

In this stage of osteoporosis prevention, hormone replacement therapy (HRT) has garnered attention since estrogen is essential for preserving bone density. HRT risks and benefits, however, need to be carefully balanced, taking into account each person's unique health circumstances and possible side effects. Other options for managing postmenopausal osteoporosis include non-hormonal interventions like selective estrogen receptor modulators (SERMs) and bisphosphonates. Modifications to lifestyle, such as an emphasis on diet and exercise, continue to be essential parts of comprehensive strategies to lessen the effects of hormone fluctuations on bone health.

a comprehensive strategy for treating and preventing osteoporosis takes into account the unique requirements and difficulties that come with each developmental stage throughout the course of a person's lifetime.

A comprehensive method to prevent osteoporosis involves promoting bone health education, encouraging healthy lifestyle practices, and including medicinal therapies as needed.

It is important to include these strategies in public health campaigns and healthcare policies to lower the incidence of fractures caused by osteoporosis and improve people's quality of life in general, regardless of their age.

CHAPTER TEN
CASE STUDIES AND SUCCESS STORIES
Individual Accounts Of Preventing Osteoporosis

Globally, osteoporosis is a major public health concern due to its frequent skeletal condition that is defined by low bone mass and microarchitectural degradation of bone tissue. Personal accounts serve as potent evidence of the effectiveness of holistic methods for treating and preventing osteoporosis while the medical profession continues to investigate them.

People who have effectively avoided or treated osteoporosis with a holistic approach frequently had similar experiences. These anecdotes add to the expanding corpus of research demonstrating the efficacy of holistic techniques and offer insightful perspectives on their practical implementation.

An ongoing motif in anecdotal tales of osteoporosis prevention is the significance of food and nutrition. Many people credit a well-balanced diet high in vital minerals like calcium, vitamin D, magnesium, and phosphorus for their ability to maintain robust bone health. These first-hand stories emphasize how crucial it is to have a range of foods high in calcium, such as dairy, fish, nuts, and leafy greens, in one's regular meals. People who take a holistic approach to eating not only take care of their urgent need for bone support but also improve their general health and wellbeing.

In addition, physical activity and exercise are essential components of individual osteoporosis prevention tales. Individuals who have successfully maintained their bone health frequently have a history of participating in strength training, flexibility training, and weight-bearing exercises. These tales highlight how important it is to engage in regular exercise to maintain bone density, strength, and resilience.

Recognizing the connection between physical health and overall well-being, holistic methods for osteoporosis prevention encourage people to follow a comprehensive exercise regimen catered to their unique requirements and preferences.

Moreover, the stories of those who have successfully avoided osteoporosis highlight stress management as a crucial element. Since long-term stress has been connected to bone loss, holistic methods place a high value on reducing stress with methods like yoga, meditation, and mindfulness. Anecdotes from personal experience show how integrating stress-reduction techniques into everyday life benefits mental and emotional wellness in addition to bone health. By addressing the complex facets of health, people may lay the groundwork for long-term prevention of osteoporosis.

Applications Of Holistic Methods In The Real World

Beyond autobiographical tales, practical implementations of holistic methods for osteoporosis prevention offer tangible illustrations of how these tactics might be applied in a variety of contexts. Policymakers, community organizations, and healthcare professionals are crucial in converting holistic ideas into practical programs that support bone health more widely. Analyzing these practical uses provides insightful information on the viability, difficulties, and achievements of applying holistic methods in many settings.

In clinical settings, medical professionals are beginning to understand how critical it is to approach osteoporosis from a holistic standpoint. Integrative care models—which blend alternative and traditional therapies—are becoming more and more popular. Examples from real-world settings demonstrate how healthcare teams work together to create individualized treatment regimens that include physical therapy, dietary counseling, and stress reduction techniques.

These multifaceted methods provide more thorough and long-lasting results for patients by addressing the underlying causes of osteoporosis in addition to bone health.

Initiatives from the community serve as additional evidence of the applicability of comprehensive strategies for osteoporosis prevention. Support groups, educational initiatives, and public health campaigns all help to increase public knowledge of the influence of lifestyle choices on bone health. Applications from everyday life demonstrate how communities work together to develop spaces that encourage exercise, easy access to wholesome meals, and tools for reducing stress.

These programs recognize that social issues impact individual health outcomes and stress the need for a community-wide effort to prevent osteoporosis.

Furthermore, by putting evidence-based solutions into practice, policymakers have a significant impact on how osteoporosis prevention is shaped. Legislative initiatives that support bone-friendly settings, such as walkability-promoting urban design and the provision of public places for leisure activities, are shown in real-world instances.

 The incorporation of holistic concepts into public health policies helps policymakers build a foundation of support for osteoporosis prevention on a large scale.

a thorough grasp of the holistic ways to manage and prevent osteoporosis is provided by the examination of individual tales and practical applications. These stories not only demonstrate the benefits of practices like stress reduction, exercise, and diet, but they also show the necessity of a multifaceted, team-based approach to bone health. To address the various elements that affect bone health and strive toward a future where osteoporosis is mitigated via a holistic lens, society may incorporate holistic concepts into clinical treatment, community initiatives, and public health regulations.

CONCLUSION

the holistic methods of managing and preventing osteoporosis, it is clear that a thorough and multidimensional strategy is necessary.

The synergistic nature of therapies that address the dietary, physical, hormonal, psychological, environmental, and lifestyle elements of bone health is highlighted in the summary of a holistic approach. One key theme that emerges is empowering people to take control of their bone health by promoting proactive involvement in preventative interventions and lifestyle adjustments. The result of these comprehensive efforts improves bone strength and density while also enhancing general health and quality of life.

A holistic viewpoint provides a strong framework for an all-encompassing and patient-centered approach to bone health as we traverse the difficulties of osteoporosis.